Vivre à Jamais

How to get a beautiful body and complexion using ancient herbs

The information in this book regarding supplements and support products is meant to be educational and is not intended to diagnose, treat, cure, or prevent disease. But if you have a serious medical condition, always consult your health-care provider The FDA has not evaluated the products in this book.

With the remedies shared in this book, you can get a healthy body and beautiful, natural, clear, healthy skin.

I would like to start with a quote from a book I wrote in 2009 about the miracle of anti-aging:

I can hear the women who epitomize women, saying we are more than just childbearing animals, from Christine de Pizan to Simone de Beauvior to Virginia Woolf to Elizabeth Lady Stanton to Susan B. Anthony to Carol Hanisch to Sara Evans to all at the UN's Pan Pacific Southeast Asia Women's Association.

Challenge the laws written in stone, even the genetic code. Everything in an exploding universe is susceptible to change and can be changed. Here we bury Hegel in a stagnant abyss, and move on.

As a woman, you will radiate a nebula of youth and beauty to be unquestioned.

The herbs we're about to talk about have been used successfully for hundreds of years by people all over the world. I'm not going to write a history of safe, beneficial skin and body herbs of the world; if you're in doubt, you can do the research.

Let's start with herbal remedies for psoriasis,

eczema, herpes, acne, blemishes, and skin diseases of all kinds, including cancer.

For a variety of skin problems, the following herbs are beneficial:

- **Burdock root**: Take capsules, 1 gram, three times per day. Safe at recommended doses.
- **Red clover**: Take two capsules, 2 grams, per day. Safe at recommended doses.
- **Dandelion root**: Take one capsule, 525mg, per day. Do not use if you have gallstones or stomach ulcers, or if you get an allergic rash. Safe at recommended doses.
- **Zinc**: Take 50mg plus 3mg of copper. Large doses of vitamin C and zinc can deplete the body of copper. Take zinc that includes copper in the formulation. Whenever you take zinc or a lot of vitamin C, you need to take a copper supplement. Safe at recommended dosages.
- **Vitamin A**: Take 25,000 IU per day. More than 25,000 IU of vitamin A can cause problems, liver damage, bone problems, and hair loss. Safe at recommended dosages.

For external use, use maximum-strength Cortizone-10 for skin inflammation, rashes, and anti-itch.

Put garlic oil on a blemish or tape a bit of real garlic over the blemish or pimple to neutralize the bacteria that is causing the problem.

Take all the vitamins and herbs together every morning with breakfast. These should clear most skin problems.

There is no cure for the herpes virus. Viruses have a habit of mimicking (disguising themselves) so that the immune system cannot recognize them (the list includes herpes, HIV, and smallpox, to name a few). To keep the virus in hibernation and prevent breakouts on your skin, you need to control stress. Stress will weaken your immune system and allow the virus to break out.

For stress, these herbs are effective:

- **Valerian root extract**: Take one 500mg capsule at night and a cup of valerian root tea in the morning and afternoon.
- **L-Lysine**: Take 500mg two times per day to inhibit the herpes virus or any virus. Take one at night and one in the morning. Safe at recommended doses.

For warts, use celandine juice or gel externally. Can be used on warts, pimples, corns, calluses, and blisters, every day, until they go away. Safe when used as recommended.

Warts are caused by a virus, HPV

(papillomavirus), and can be found almost everywhere.

In modern medicine, there is no cure for cancer.

I like to think of modern medicine as a medieval medicine, considering the way doctors cut, burn, drug, and put contraptions in human bodies that never work for the love of money.

For cancer, take graviola caplets, 3,000mg, two times per day. You can buy organic freeze-dried graviola on the Internet.

Eat fifteen apricots kernels three times per day. You can buy organic apricot kernels on the Internet.

Drink a lot of chaga tea. You can buy organic chaga tea at www.chagamountain.com.

Take as many vitamin C capsules as you can, from 1,000mg to 10,000mg, three times per day.

Again, it is all about the folk medicine that has been used for thousands of years all over planet Earth. If you want to know more, you can do the research. This book is about you being beautiful and having a beautiful body.

Let us move on.

Teas—you should drink tea often. There is no specific amount of each, but drink one every day.

Beneficial teas for skin and body, which make

you look and feel better, will do more good than that cup of coffee that gets you going in the morning and damages your skin and your body.

In the morning with breakfast and throughout the day, drink:

- Organic burdock root tea
- Organic red clover tea
- Organic roasted dandelion tea
- Organic green tea
- Organic valerian root tea
- Organic ashwagandha root tea

Even better, mix them together and drink them. You can buy the teas at www.buddhateas.com. Take the pills and drink the teas; you will have a beautiful complexion.

Sounds simple, right? Just drink a few teas and give up the coffee. There is a lot of magic in herbal pills and teas to promote healthy, beautiful skin.

You may be noticing that you are starting to look and feel better, and blemishes and some wrinkles are disappearing.

There is more you need to do to be beautiful. You can buy these two products online at www. iherb.com (Reviva Labs): DMAE firming fluid (1fl oz) and Alpha Lipoic Acid, Vitamin C Ester, and DMAE cream. Apply to wrinkles, sagging skin, and neck—whatever part of your body needs attention—

every night before bed. Try it on your lips for a fuller appearance before you go out.

If you have come this far, you can see the changes. A healthy, beautiful body and a beautiful complexion can be yours. Now that you are starting to get a beautiful complexion, let us work on that beautiful body.

A beautiful body requires a healthy body. These herbs will help you achieve optimal health:

Wild Mexican yam extract root: Take 300mg capsules or tablets of the dried root, one capsule per day. Used for hundreds of years in folk medicine—East Indian, Chinese, and American—to treat painful menstruation, asthma, fatigue, and cramps. Side effects: some people get nausea when taking large amounts. Safe at recommended doses.

Vitamin C: At night before bed, take a vitamin C time-release tablet, 1,000mg per day. Vitamin C makes collagen in the body, promotes healing, and supports liver function. The more you take, the better—just know that large doses will deplete copper in the body, so if you take 5,000mg or 10,000mg per day, supplement with copper.

DMAE (dimethylaminoethanol): Take one capsule, 100mg, per day. Can tighten and tone the skin and reduce the buildup of skin pigmentation caused by aging. Safe in recommended doses.

Alpha Lipoic Acid: Take one time-release tablet, 300mg per day. Will neutralize free radical damage. Safe at recommended dosages.

Natural vitamin E, pure D-alpha: Take two 400 IU softgels per day. Provides antioxidants that will benefit the body, prevent most diseases, and help heal all conditions. Safe; no known side effects.

Vitamin C Ester: Take 500mg per day. Promotes anti-aging; treats uneven skin tone, loss of firmness, and wrinkles; and supports natural collagen production.

CoQ10: Take 30 mg per day. CoQ10 is part of the energy production of every cell in the human body. Safe; if you have a heart condition and are taking large doses, you should not discontinue without talking to your doctor.

Selenium: Take 200mg per day. Activates thyroid hormones; prevents cancer.

Calcium plus vitamin D: For preventing osteoporosis, rickets, migraine headaches, and more. Nature's Bounty absorbable calcium with vitamin D3 contains calcium (1,000mg) and vitamin D (100 IU). Safe at recommended doses.

Bilberry extract: Take 240mg per day. Prevents cataracts; promotes healthy eyes. No known side effects.

Glucosamine sulfate: Take 1,000mg per day. Promotes the repair of bones and cartilage. Safe; no known side effects. (Some glucosamine sulfate may be processed with table salt. If you have high blood pressure, make sure it's not processed with sodium chloride.)

Omega-3 fish oil: Take 1,000mg per day. Anti-inflammatory; prevents heart disease. High levels of vitamin D and vitamin A. Do not take cod liver oil. Safe at recommended doses.

Vitamin B6: Take 100mg per day. Essential healing for carpal tunnel syndrome and many diseases. Needed to process amino acids in the body. Safe at recommended doses; very high levels of over 500mg can cause damage to sensory nerves.

Garlic: Take one 1,000mg capsule per day. Everyone knows what good things garlic can do for you. It has been around for thousands of years. It's beneficial to conditions of high cholesterol, atherosclerosis, and congestive heart failure and provides immune support. Because of garlic's anticlotting effect, if you're taking anticoagulant drugs, check with your doctor before taking garlic. No known side effects.

Grapeseed extract: Take one 300mg capsule per day. May prevent skin cancer; treats heart disease and macular degeneration. Safe; no known side effects.

Dandelion root: Take 525mg, one per day. Used for hundreds of years to treat liver and kidney disease, eczema, and health problems like alcoholism. Works as a blood purifier. Safe, but persons with gallstones or stomach ulcers should not take dandelion. In some people, it may cause an allergic rash.

Alfalfa: Buy Alfa-max, by Nature's Way; take 525mg, three capsules at night. Used for thousands of years in China and India and by American Indians to treat arthritis, water retention, problems with digestion, anemia, and diabetes, and to prevent hardening of the arteries. Safe at recommended doses; there are isolated reports of persons allergic to alfalfa.

Evening Primrose oil: Take 1,000mg per day. If you have cysts, take 4,000 per day for four weeks; the cysts should be gone. For healthier skin and hair. Safe; no known side effects (drink only distilled water).

Eat only fresh USA organic meat, fish, fruits, and vegetables—no frozen or processed organic food.

Exercise is important, but why knock yourself out? All the exercise you need is in a tai chi class—it is like slow dancing with health benefits.

One half hour before you work out, take BCAAs (Branched-Chain Amino Acids). Take three capsules. You can buy them at your vitamin store. BCAAs help athletic performance and reduce muscle loss. There are no known side effects. This amino acid is converted in the body and used as energy.

You are never too old or too young to be beautiful and healthy. Now you know what you have to do to get beautiful skin and a beautiful body; do it.

If you are fifty years or older, we need to talk about menopause.

There are different types of hormone replacement therapy; all of them have side effects ranging from heart disease to a high risk of cancer.

Herbal remedies are better. These include:

Black Cohosh: Standardized extracts are available with 1mg of deoxyactein per tablet. Take 40mg twice per day for six months. Do not use if pregnant. Side effects: large doses may cause nausea, headaches, dizziness, or abdominal pain; if you are on estrogen, consult your physician.

Vitex: You can buy Nature's Way Vitex 400mg; take one capsule three times per day for five or six months, then one per day. Side effects are rare. Mild itching occurs in 2 percent of women taking Vitex.

St. John's Wort: Take 500mg per day, tablets or capsules. Safe in recommended doses. Not to be used during pregnancy. High doses make skin more light sensitive; you should not be exposed to strong sunlight at any time anyway. It can damage your skin. It is not advisable to drink alcohol when taking

St. John's wort.

Kava: Take 210mg of kava-lactones per day. Side effects: at recommended doses, mild gastrointestinal disturbances may occur in some people. Do not take high dosages of kava; it may turn skin yellow. Not recommended for pregnant or lactating women. Should not be taken with alcohol or any substances like barbiturates or antidepressants.

GABA (gamma-aminobutyric acid): Take one 750mg dose at night. An inhibitory neurotransmitter that calms the mind.

If you still have problems such as fatigue, low energy, or anxiety, have your doctor check you for hypothyroidism. The therapy is thyroxin.

Whatever you are prescribed, start with a low dose of 25mg. If it works for you, stay with it; if not, gradually increase the dose until it works. Stay with whatever works for you.

There is no such thing one size fits all, not when it comes to humans. Human reactions to all things are different.

You may not be in menopause.

And if you think you can get all of this from the food you eat, that may have been the case seventy years ago; today, with soil that has little or no nutritional value, and food processing and trucking, the food you eat has no nutritional value.

The problem of wrinkles or sagging skin has to do with the problem of aging, and the problem of aging is that in gerontology there is no universal aging theory; there are a number of hypotheses. These include developmental, genetic, the Hayflick limit, error, cross-linkage, energy restriction, free radical, and autoimmune, to name a few, and my theory, the dispersing atoms theory. We will talk about all these.

Then there is pathologic aging (aging caused by disease).

If you have a disease, you need to address the cause of the disease. Your doctor will treat the symptom, but the problem will never go away. But if you find the cause and eliminate it, the problem goes away and your doctor will say you're in remission, because doctors are not trained to find the cause of a disease. They are trained to name everything a disease. As you live your life, your body will produce all kinds of abnormalities that are held in check and never affect your health. Tumors that are found in your body after you are dead are called incidentalomas. Your doctor will test you and find problems that can lead to unjustifiable surgery and treatment that will do more damage than good. This book can help you eliminate the cause of disease.

A disease can fast-forward aging in humans. If your doctor has wrinkles, do not listen to him about how he can help you when he cannot help himself.

If he says "it is in your genes," he has no clue. Today we know the genome is not a permanent record of life and that in fact, the genome is a living organ that can adapt and change. Under stress, genes can move and influence other genes and create change, a process called "jumping genes."

The study of epigenetics and the Human Epigenome Project in time will give us a better understanding from our birth to what we are and why we are aging.

There is no magic pill, no magic cream: we live in a complex world parasitized by a retrovirus.

That gives us intellect. Viruses are genetic creators. Sound strange? It may take another book to explain. Viruses can change and create animal behavior, like the rabies virus. Women that are infected with the parasite T. gondii (toxoplasma gondii) are "easy"—they have more relationships with men. The common cold that will not kill you will just keep you well enough to run around coughing and sneezing on everyone.

We live in a place where our skin is affected by viruses, bacteria, and damage caused by carcinogens and nitrates in our food, tobacco smoke, alcohol, pesticides, insecticides, fumes, aerosol sprays, fluoride, and so much more.

Avoiding and neutralizing all of this is a way to

have beautiful skin and a beautiful body. You need to affect your complex body chemistry with a remedy that is complex and that can interact in a good way and give you what you want. That's why you take a lot of different vitamins and nutrients that all work together to make you look and feel beautiful. Taking one pill, or undergoing one procedure, will never work because your skin is an organ; like your heart, lungs, etc., it interacts with your whole body. It protects it, holds it together, and what you put in your body and what you put on your body will have an effect, good or bad, and strengthen or weaken your skin. If you have skin problems, you need to strengthen your skin not only externally, but internally as well.

Your skin, like your whole body, is interactive. This may not sound right to you because we live in a world where doctors tell us we are a lot of parts. When some parts are not working, they send you to a specialist that can fix the broken part. It never works, so then they send you to another specialist and on and on, and your body rejects the repaired part.

Humans are not made of parts; the whole human body is connected. That is how you can walk across a street, drive a car, play music—you do all these things with your whole body, not with just one part. In the real world, people use their whole bodies to do everything they do.

If you live in a stressful life with a grin on your face, it will affect your whole body. You cannot fix your skin and not change the way you think, eat, and live. Your doctor cannot fix your skin with medicine or plastic surgery. You have to fix your mind and body, not only from the outside but from the inside—from what you eat to the way you think, from the air you are breathing to the environment you are living in, everything has an effect on your skin. Some people cannot get away from stress. There are people in our lives that stress us out all the time. You may be thinking you have to live with stress. If you accept it and live with stress, it will make you old, wrinkled, and diseased.

For stress that you have to live with, take:

- 500mg valerian root herbal extract in capsules one hour before bed
- One cup of valerian root tea before work and a cup at work
- Kava capsules
- A cup of kava tea before bed
- GABA to calm your mind.

Let comedy be a part of your everyday life. Watch TV shows that make you laugh. Go to comedy shows, tell jokes, make fun of the people that stress you out; the joy and laughter will resonate through your whole body and make you a healthier, happier person.

You will look beautiful; people will ask why you are always happy and laughing all the time. Tell them, "It makes me beautiful and healthy—you should try it."

Take the fake grin off your face and get those smiley muscles working. After a while, it will become a permanent look. You will look happy, and if you look happy, feel happy, and act happy, you will be happy (a bit of Confucian philosophy).

Why some people look and feel angry most of the time

I hope no one reading what I'm about to say feels I am targeting any specific people or group. Given the science of epigenetics, we now know that genes under environmental stress can move and change the code of other genes and change what you are. These jumping genes become part of the DNA of an organism and change the encoded sequence, and now you have an angry gene, radical gene, passive gene, etc., that is passed on for generations.

After hundreds of years of Islamic radicalism, their offspring are born with a radical gene, and we know what they are doing today. The offspring of American slaves are born with an anger gene and are filling all the jails of America. Tribes of American

Indians, after fighting other tribes for a hundred years, have a violent gene. Their offspring today are finding it hard to control their violent impulses and are getting into all kinds of trouble.

On the flip side, groups of people that have lived a passive, well-mannered life for hundreds, even thousands of years, have a passive gene. Some of these communities include the offspring of the Zen (their communities are calm and settled) and the offspring of the Buddhists (they would not hurt a fly).

What has this got to do with beautiful skin? It has everything to do with it. You have to understand your emotions and what makes you what you are, and have the courage to take whatever steps you must to block the effect of those genes and create a calm mental state, or it will affect your whole body. Treating stress with the methods explained in this book is a good start.

There is a lot more that makes you what you are and influences how you behave. It was nice, back in the day, when B. F. Skinner had us all believing that positive reinforcement theory can change anyone and turn bad behavior into good behavior. Then good old Gestalt proved him wrong.

Do not ask me to explain Gestalt therapy or behaviorism—trust me, some things stay with us for hundreds of years.

A lot of people take over-the-counter drugs and prescription drugs. Most of the drugs you are taking are chelating—that is, they bind with minerals in the body and make them unavailable to the body. A mineral deficiency can cause real health problems. Doctors and consumers need to understand the long-term effects of prescription drugs and the nutritional deficiencies caused by drugs, which can be preventable if you and your doctor understand what minerals in your body are affected by the prescription drugs you are taking. You can supplement with the minerals that are affected and avoid having more health problems caused by a side effect your doctor is not aware of.

Humans are complex animals and change is always an event in our lives; take, for example, cross-species transference.

If what you and your family have been eating for the last twenty or more years is mostly chicken, you are high-energy, with a pecking order mentally. You are striving to move up in the social order of our society. Perhaps you even look like a chicken.

If you have been eating mostly beef, you need to be part of a group (the herd mentality). Maybe you are even a wide-eyed, big person (like a cow).

What you have been eating is important, and what you will eat from now on is more important.

The saying is "you are what you eat." It's more

like what you feel, look, and act like comes from what you eat. It's all part of being beautiful.

This parasitic idea can turn anyone off. No one likes parasites, and I would like to quote from a book I wrote in 2009:

> Humans are the macro parasites of planet Earth. In their existence, humans have driven into extinction countless numbers of life forms. Humans are capable of killing off their own species. Humans move in groups, interacting with other groups of their own species, trading goods, maintaining border patrols, protecting boundaries, attacking neighbors, and using pure, natural animal instincts. Their leadership phenomenon is natural in the entire animal world; the consumption of alcohol and other drugs throughout history accounts for humans' abnormal behavior. The drugs and chemicals humans consume today have evolved. The effects are new abnormal behaviors and diseases.

> The fact of the matter is that you are part of an animal herd roaming the earth. Just because you are reading this book means nothing. It cannot change what you are, what you are doing on this planet, or the effect you have on this planet. It is because you are a parasite that you have managed to come this far.

Your technology is from the aftermath of world wars and millions of humans killed—the jet plane, the rocket, the atomic bomb, industrial farming. The killing of plant and animal life for a few good crops and meat.

That was in 2009; today I know it's a proven scientific fact that parasitic viruses and the food we eat can change human behavior. How smart can humans be if a parasitic retrovirus is regulating human life, and we look and behave like the animals we eat?

Let us get back to being beautiful.

Use a natural soap that is kind to your skin, one that works with your skin and does not cause damage to sensitive, delicate skin. Grisi Chamomile is one.

Chamomile has a healing effect on skin. Chamomile tea is good for your skin. Drink it and put the tea on your skin. The Kiss My Face products are soaps you may want to try.

If you have oily skin, your natural oil protects your skin so do not overwash your face. Use a mild natural cleanser formulated for oily or combination skin that will remove makeup without drying skin in the morning and at night before bed.

You do not need all those different products that are supposed to make you look like Cleopatra. Do not waste your money.

If you must be out in the sun, you will need a good natural sunscreen. It's best not to be out in the sun.

Again, eat only USA organic foods, and no sugar of any kind, especially refined white sugar. No salt.

You can use honey to sweeten whatever you wish. Salt and sugar will destroy your skin and cause wrinkles.

Try not to eat a lot of meat; if you must, let be it USA organic.

Organic fruits and vegetables are good, but organic frozen and processed food is a problem because it's cooked in partially hydrogenated vegetable oil. Even when the label says zero trans fats, there is no other way it can stay fresh for months or years in the freezer.

Yes, fresh for six months or a year—TFAs (trans-fatty acids) are poison. Over time they get into cells and disrupt the integrity of cell membranes and walls, causing health problems that affect the whole body.

Read labels. If the ingredient list says partially hydrogenated, the product has trans fats.

TFAs will give you wrinkles, sagging skin, and many diseases you do not want, including cancer.

Most restaurants use hydrogenated oils to cook their food; it costs a lot less, foods last longer, and they do not need to change the oil; they can cook in the same oil forever. It will not get rancid.

It's a good reason to cook everything in olive oil. Cooking with electricity in stainless steel pots is healthier.

Some things that cause skin damage include sun exposure, stress, free radicals in the environment, toxins in tap water, harmful chemicals in food and drinks, excess cigarette smoke, and alcohol. Your immune system's inability to deal with all or any of this causes the dermis cells lose their ability to rebuild the collagen that holds all of it together. You will get sagging, dry skin and start to see wrinkles. You're thinking you're getting old and that's what happens when you get old. That's not what is happening. When you look at a baby's skin, it is beautiful and wrinkle free. The baby's body is replacing the epidermis (the skin's outer layer), and the dermis (under the epidermis) that produces oil, perspiration, and collagen is holding it all together and chemically keeping it all in a natural balance. And under it all is a fat layer that protects the body and gives the baby that plump look.

It is all working the same as it was when you were a baby, except today there are some things that are disrupting the system and turning off essential hormones, which weakens the immune system. But can you get everything working as it was when you were a baby and have beautiful skin?

That baby has an abundance of growth hormone, which creates beautiful skin and a beautiful body and a strong immune system, yet it's just beginning to be exposed to the toxic environment we live in, it is just starting to eat the toxic food we eat, and it is just beginning to become stressed out from the neglect.

It can deal with all of the damage caused by all of this because it has a strong immune system.

One day when you are forty-five to fifty years old, the support that your immune system needs is turned off. From that day on, your body is affected by all things that damage human cells, and the process of human aging begins.

You think all you can do is plastic surgery; again, that's your doctor trying to fix parts. You are thinking wrong. You are not fooling anyone. Everyone knows what plastic surgery looks like. In addition, in time it all falls apart because you are not addressing the cause. Your doctor is addressing the symptoms.

Understand the cause, and if you cannot avoid all the things that cause aging, then neutralize what you have to be exposed to, like car fumes. It's the way to beautiful skin.

If you have come this far and are doing some of the things we have talked about, you are beginning to look beautiful.

However, we still need to understand the hypotheses of aging.

Developmental: the idea that some people are fifty and look seventy, and some are seventy and look fifty because of lifestyle, diseases, etc.—no one is sure of the cause.

Genetic Theories

The Hayflick Limit Theory

Cells regenerate so many times grown in a culture medium and then die of cause; no consideration for improper functioning of cells in the real world. An experiment in isolation. Humans are an integrative species, not something that grows in a petri dish.

Error Theory

The idea that a catastrophe happens and causes a cascade of effects. Not all cells accumulate misspecified molecules. In addition, aging is not accelerated when this happens.

Redundant DNA Theory

Like the error theory but with genes; it cannot explain normal aging factors, radiation-induced aging, and other aspects of aging.

The Wear-Tear Theory

Like a machine, the body wears out, then you get diseases. This theory does not explain anything; it just equates humans to machines, so like a machine, things break down. Sounds good, but we are not machines.

Cross-Linkage Theory

The idea that collagen breaks down due to cross-linkage of DNA. Two molecules become cross-linked, causing damage to the collagen and deeper layers of the skin. The cause may be free radicals, exposure to solar radiation, everything from food to environmental agents.

There is a lot to say about this theory and the idea that one can take antioxidants, vitamins, and nutrients as effective inhibitors to prevent damaging cross-linkage reactions.

Autoimmune Theory

In time, the immune system gets weaker and cannot stop diseases and whatever attacks the body, which it had no problem dealing with when you were young. It does not explain *why* the immune system fails with age and why all older people do not get autoimmune disease.

The Rate of Living Theory

Everyone has a limited amount of time or energy in a world where energy, over time, is depleted. No one knows what this energy is or that it even exists.

Free Radical Theory

Highly charged ions damage cell membranes through a reaction called lipid peroxidation. An accumulation of age pigment (called lipofuscin, not the dark-brown spots on one's face) in lysosomes can be seen at microscopic levels in the tissues of the body. Oxygen and nutrient supplies are blocked, causing the death of tissue.

Hormonal Theory

The brain is were Aging begins the ability of the pituitary gland that controls the thyroid gland it's secretion of thyroxin the master rate-controlling hormone within the body. The problem is the antiaging serum has not been found. Alternatively, there is no satisfactory evidence, because menopause is a hormone event, and does not regulate aging.

I would like to add to this that retroviruses are made of RNA, and RNA is a greater part of brain chemistry and has the ability to change brain DNA, giving humans problem-solving abilities to populate the world, insuring the parasites' survival and placing an aging factor in human DNA to ensure that humans do not overpopulate like the common cold virus that will not kill you and lets you walk and spread the flu.

This virus regulates human life. One may call it the theory of parasites.

Another theory of mind, the disbursing atoms, needs no explanation. We are all made of atoms; atoms move about and crash into one another, and atoms are lost.

Your whole body is interactive and if you go to your doctor and get replacement parts that are not biological, interactive parts, it will not work. The parts will fall apart, and you will be in worse shape. Everyone knows that. Then what?

Of human biological complexities, human neurochemistry, human electrical chemistry, and the balancing act of all this collectively working together in billions of interactions every second of your life, your doctor has not the vaguest idea; no one has.

If you are a healthy person, then you should have healthier skin.

OK, then what? Let's start with what you should eat. Eat the food you like, yes, but most of the food you eat is made to taste good by food companies adding sugar and salt and artificial flavors. They make it taste good and look good, and in time it will kill you. It may be better to eat the food your ancestors ate because you are more genetically inclined to that food (epigenetic) and it may be healthier for you. Your ancestors did not live in the chemical invasion epoch we live in today; their food did not have the chemicals that damage your immune system and speed the onslaught of sagging and wrinkled skin. You still can eat your ancestors' food, just a USA organic version—no salt, no refined sugar, no processed food, no frozen food. Eat lots of USA organic fruits and vegetables and brown rice, and drink lots of distilled water. Cook fresh fish a few times a week, assuming your ancestors were eating such food. What your grandparents were eating and what they were drinking has an effect on what you are and the way you behave. It was passed down through your parents to you.

I will assume you're eating the right foods and taking the right pills. Today we cannot stop the human aging process, but we can slow it down to a crawl. In addition, you can look beautiful and be healthy in the process.

About the age of fifty, your brain tells your body to stop the body's production of growth hormone, which is released from your pituitary gland when you sleep or exercise. The retrovirus that is part of your DNA turns off the switch, and the production of growth hormone stops.

Growth hormone improves your immune system and helps fight disease, converts fat into muscle, helps tissue repair, and gives you a healthier, youthful body. It is what makes young people young.

When the release of growth hormone in the human body stops, the process that activates and promotes the aging process begins.

One of the things that the virus, which is part of human DNA, may be doing is regulating human life so that we do not overpopulate the planet.

This virus may also affect human behavior, making us go to war and kill off one another en masse. We need not concern ourselves with such theories.

We can do nothing about war, but we can take amino acids that stimulate the pituitary gland and release growth hormone in our bodies when we sleep. They will give a youthful body and slow the aging process.

To stimulate the production of growth hormone in the body, you need to take amino acids at night before bed on an empty stomach with water and no protein:

- **L-Ornithine:** 1,000mg per day
- **L-Arginine:** 500mg per day (if you have the herpes virus, take L-Arginine one time a week)
- **Glycine:** 500mg per day
- **Tryptophan:** 1,000mg per day

- **Tyrosine:** 1,000mg per day
- **L- Lysine:** 1,000mg per day

The amino acids work better with the supplements. Take vitamins C and B6 and a multiple mineral with magnesium, zinc, and calcium.

Replacing the growth hormone that made you look young when you were young will generate a youthful biological condition.

Can't remember things? Take ginkgo. Take it every day. You will remember things in a short time.

The feedback aspect

There is one more aspect of all of this. We now understand that as humans we are an interacting entity affected by our environment: what we eat, how we live, what we see, what we feel, and the way we think about ourselves and aging, all combine to give us feedback.

To make all of this work, you need to control the feedback you're getting, which is creating the person you want to be.

First, you have to look young to yourself. This means no gray hair; gray hair sends signals to your body that it's time for you to be old. You control what you are and it's not time to be old, so get rid of all the gray hair. It is better to not have any hair than to have gray hair.

Life is just beginning for you. Spend your money on yourself. It's not too late to create an active mind.

Yes, take that music class you always wanted to but did not have the time for—today, make the time for it. You have a life to live.

Yes, take that tai chi class. It's great exercise, and again it is like slow dancing with health benefits.

Yes, look in the mirror and say to yourself, "I look younger, I feel younger, and with all the things I am doing, I am more beautiful than I have ever been in all my life." Say it every day. If you do everything in this book, you will feel it because you will be beautiful and have a beautiful body. That is the feedback aspect.

You look beautiful and think beautiful, and if you look and think beautiful, you are beautiful and you will stay beautiful and have a beautiful body, and everyone will love you; it's all part of being beautiful.

Keep in mind

Most doctors are invested in the diagnostic centers that they refer their patients to for testing. Doctors and the pharmaceutical industry need to create diseases to sell prescription drugs. That is how they make a living. Don't get caught up in the high cholesterol or high blood pressure hysteria; you may be treated for a condition you don't have. Doctors selling drugs and tests make a very nice living, but that living can prove harmful to you.

Stay beautiful: vivre à jamais.